CHAIR YOGA FOR WEIGHT LOSS

A Step-by-Step Guide to Shedding Pounds, Boosting Energy, and Embracing Wellness for Seniors and Beginners

Smith Bami

CONTENTS

WELCOME TO CHAIR YOGA FOR WEIGHT LOSS

Are you ready to embark on a journey that will not only reshape your body but also rejuvenate your spirit and uplift your mind? If so, you've come to the right place. Allow me to extend a warm and heartfelt welcome as you begin this transformative experience with chair yoga.

Now, you might be wondering, what exactly is chair yoga, and how can it help you achieve your weight loss goals? Well, let me tell you: chair yoga is not just your average workout routine. It's a gentle yet powerful practice that combines the ancient wisdom of yoga with the accessibility of a chair, making it suitable for people of all ages, abilities, and fitness levels. And in this book, we're going to explore how chair yoga can be your secret weapon in the battle against unwanted pounds.

But before we dive into the nitty-gritty details, let's talk about why you're here and what you can expect to gain from this book. You see, I believe that weight loss is not just about shedding pounds on the scale; it's about transforming your entire being from the inside out. It's about reclaiming your confidence, embracing your body, and nurturing your soul. And that's exactly what chair yoga can help you achieve.

Inside these pages, you'll discover a treasure trove of chair yoga poses specifically curated to target those stubborn areas where excess weight tends to linger. From gentle stretches to dynamic flows, each pose is designed to activate your muscles, boost your metabolism, and ignite your inner fire—all from the comfort of your favorite chair. But that's not all. You'll also learn how to harness the power of breath, mindfulness, and self-love to supercharge your weight loss journey and create lasting change from the inside out.

But perhaps most importantly, this book is about empowering you to become the best version of yourself—not just physically, but emotionally and spiritually as well. It's about embracing your unique journey, celebrating your progress, and finding joy in every step along the way. So if you're ready to say goodbye to crash diets, punishing workouts, and self-doubt, and hello to a healthier, happier you, then I invite you to join me on this transformative adventure.

Are you ready to unlock the secrets of chair yoga for weight loss? Then let's embark on this journey together. Your body, mind, and spirit will thank you.

Welcome aboard!

BENEFITS OF CHAIR YOGA FOR WEIGHT LOSS

Welcome to the heart of our journey—where we unveil the remarkable benefits of chair yoga for shedding those unwanted pounds and sculpting the body of your dreams. Are you ready to discover how a gentle, seated practice can ignite your metabolism, tone your muscles, and unleash your inner strength? Let's dive in!

1. **Accessible for All**: One of the most beautiful aspects of chair yoga is its inclusivity. Regardless of age, fitness level, or physical ability, everyone can reap the rewards of this practice. Whether you're a seasoned yogi or a complete newbie, the supportive framework of the chair provides a stable foundation for exploring movement, breath, and mindfulness—all essential components of a successful weight loss journey.

2. **Gentle Yet Effective**: Say goodbye to grueling workouts that leave you feeling depleted and

discouraged. Chair yoga offers a kinder, gentler approach to fitness that honors your body's unique needs and limitations. By moving mindfully and with intention, you can activate dormant muscles, improve circulation, and stimulate your metabolism—all without putting undue strain on your joints or risking injury.

3. **Boosts Metabolism**: Did you know that certain yoga poses can actually rev up your metabolism and enhance calorie burning? It's true! Through a combination of dynamic movements, deep breathing, and mindful awareness, chair yoga can help stoke the metabolic fires within, turning your body into a more efficient fat-burning machine. Plus, the added bonus of increased circulation means more oxygen and nutrients delivered to your cells, supporting overall health and vitality.

4. **Strengthens and Tones Muscles**: Don't let the seated nature of chair yoga fool you—this practice packs a powerful punch when it comes to building strength and sculpting lean muscle mass. From

core-engaging twists to arm-strengthening flows, each pose targets specific muscle groups, helping to tone and tighten your body from head to toe. And because you're seated throughout the practice, you can focus on proper alignment and technique without the distractions of balancing on unstable surfaces.

5. **Promotes Mindful Eating**: Weight loss isn't just about what happens on the mat—it's also about what happens off the mat, particularly in the kitchen. Chair yoga teaches us to cultivate mindfulness and awareness in all aspects of our lives, including our eating habits. By tuning into our body's hunger and fullness cues, practicing mindful eating, and savoring each bite with intention, we can break free from unhealthy patterns of overeating and emotional eating, paving the way for lasting weight loss success.

6. **Reduces Stress and Anxiety**: Let's face it—stress is a major contributor to weight gain and difficulty in losing weight. The good news? Chair yoga offers

a sanctuary of calm amidst the chaos of daily life. Through gentle stretches, soothing breathwork, and guided relaxation, you can melt away tension, calm your nervous system, and quiet the mind—a crucial step on the path to achieving your weight loss goals.

Intrigued? Inspired? I hope so! These are just a few of the many benefits that chair yoga has to offer for weight loss. So grab a chair, roll out your mat, and let's embark on this transformative journey together.

MY CHAIR YOGA FOR WEIGHT LOSS EXPERIENCE

Welcome, dear reader, to a chapter close to my heart—a chapter where vulnerability meets resilience, and where personal triumphs pave the way for shared success. As we journey together through the realm of chair yoga for weight loss, allow me to open the door to my own experience—a journey filled with challenges, setbacks, and ultimately, profound transformation.

Like many of you, my relationship with weight loss has been a rollercoaster ride—one marked by highs of determination and lows of frustration. I've tried countless diets, embarked on rigorous exercise routines, and even dabbled in trendy fads, all in pursuit of that elusive goal: a fitter, healthier me. And yet, despite my best efforts, the pounds stubbornly refused to budge, leaving me feeling defeated and disheartened.

It wasn't until I discovered chair yoga that everything changed. At first, I'll admit, I was skeptical. How could something as gentle and serene as chair yoga possibly help me achieve my weight loss goals? But as I immersed myself in the practice—exploring the depths of each pose, surrendering to the rhythm of my breath, and embracing the stillness within—I began to experience profound shifts, both physically and emotionally.

However, it wasn't all smooth sailing. I encountered obstacles along the way—moments of doubt, frustration, and even pain. There were days when my body resisted, when my mind wandered, and when the voice of self-doubt grew deafeningly loud. But through it all, I persisted. I sought guidance from experienced instructors, listened to the wisdom of my own body, and approached each challenge with an open heart and mind.

And you know what? Slowly but surely, the pieces began to fall into place. I noticed subtle changes in my body— increased flexibility, improved posture, and yes, even a few inches lost around the waistline. But more importantly, I felt a profound sense of peace and empowerment wash over me—a newfound confidence in my body's capabilities and a deep-seated trust in the wisdom of the practice.

Today, I can say with certainty that chair yoga has transformed not only my body but also my entire outlook on life. It has taught me to approach challenges with grace and resilience, to embrace the journey with curiosity and humility, and to find joy in every breath, every movement, every moment.

So to you, dear reader, I extend an invitation—a invitation to embark on this transformative journey with me. Know that you are not alone, that your struggles are valid, and that your triumphs are within reach. Together, let us embrace the practice of chair yoga with open hearts and open minds, knowing that the path to weight loss is not just about shedding pounds but also about finding joy, finding peace, and finding ourselves along the way.

Are you ready to write your own story of triumph? Then let's roll out our mats, take a seat, and dive into the transformative world of chair yoga for weight loss. Your journey begins now.

GETTING STARTED

- **Setting Achievable Weight Loss Goals Through Chair Yoga**

1. **Define Your Vision**: Close your eyes and envision the best version of yourself—the version that is strong, vibrant, and full of vitality. What does that look like? What does it feel like? Take a moment to connect with your deepest desires and aspirations, and let that vision guide you as we journey together.

2. **Set SMART Goals**: Now that you have a clear vision in mind, it's time to turn that vision into reality through the power of goal-setting. Remember the acronym SMART—Specific, Measurable, Achievable, Relevant, and Time-bound. Rather than setting vague goals like "lose weight" or "get in shape," be specific and strategic. For example, "I will practice chair yoga for 20 minutes, three times a week, for the next three months, with the goal of losing 10 pounds."

3. **Break it Down**: Rome wasn't built in a day, and neither is lasting weight loss achieved overnight. Break your larger goal into smaller, manageable steps or milestones, each one bringing you closer to your ultimate destination. Celebrate each milestone along the way, acknowledging your progress and resilience.

4. **Stay Flexible**: While it's important to set goals and create a roadmap for success, it's equally important to remain flexible and adaptable along the way. Life is unpredictable, and obstacles are bound to arise. Rather than viewing setbacks as failures, see them as opportunities for growth and learning. Adjust your course as needed, but never lose sight of your ultimate destination.

5. **Believe in Yourself**: Perhaps the most important ingredient in achieving your goals is belief—in yourself, in your abilities, and in the power of chair yoga to facilitate transformation. Remember that you are capable of more than you can imagine, and that nothing is impossible when you set your mind

to it. Cultivate a mindset of positivity, resilience, and unwavering determination, knowing that you have everything you need to succeed within you.

6. **Stay Motivated**: On days when doubt creeps in and motivation wanes, remember why you started this journey in the first place. Reconnect with your vision, revisit your goals, and draw inspiration from your own inner strength and resilience. Surround yourself with supportive friends, family, or fellow practitioners who uplift and encourage you along the way. And most importantly, never lose sight of the fact that you are capable of achieving greatness—both on and off the mat.

7. **Believe in Yourself**: Cultivate a positive mindset and believe in your ability to succeed. Remind yourself of your strengths, past accomplishments, and the progress you've already made. Trust in your capacity to overcome challenges and achieve your goals with perseverance and determination.

8. **Relevance is Key**: Your goals should align with your overall objectives and values. Make sure they

are meaningful and relevant to you, whether it's improving your health, boosting your confidence, or enhancing your overall well-being.

9. **Make Them Measurable**: Set goals that you can track and measure over time. This could include tracking your weight, measuring inches lost, or monitoring your progress in specific yoga poses.

10. **Ensure They're Achievable**: Choose goals that are challenging yet realistic for you. Consider your current fitness level, lifestyle, and any potential barriers, and set goals that you believe you can realistically achieve with dedication and effort.

• Importance Of Proper Posture And Technique In Chair Yoga Poses

As we explore the tenfold importance of mastering these foundational aspects of chair yoga, remember: attention to detail is key, and every small adjustment brings you one step closer to success.

Alignment Is Everything: Proper alignment is the cornerstone of a safe and effective chair yoga practice. Aligning your body correctly in each pose ensures that you engage the right muscles, avoid strain or injury, and maximize the benefits of the pose.

Supports Muscle Engagement: When you maintain proper posture and technique, you activate the muscles needed to support your body in each pose. This engagement not only strengthens and tones your muscles but also enhances your overall stability and balance.

Optimizes Breath and Energy Flow: Proper posture and alignment allow for optimal breath and energy flow throughout your body. By aligning your spine, opening your chest, and elongating your torso, you create space for deeper, more expansive breaths, which oxygenate your cells, invigorate your mind, and fuel your practice.

Enhances Mind-Body Connection: Paying attention to your posture and technique fosters a deeper connection between your mind and body. As you tune into the subtle sensations of each movement and adjust your alignment accordingly, you cultivate mindfulness, presence, and self-awareness—a powerful trifecta for transformative change.

Prevents Injury and Discomfort: Poor posture and alignment can lead to discomfort, strain, or even injury, undermining your progress and hindering your ability to fully engage with the practice. By prioritizing proper technique, you mitigate the risk of injury and create a safe, supportive environment for your body to thrive.

Promotes Efficient Movement Patterns: Mastering proper posture and technique allows you to move more efficiently and gracefully through each pose. By minimizing unnecessary tension or effort and moving with fluidity and ease, you conserve energy, enhance performance, and experience greater freedom of movement.

Facilitates Deeper Stretching and Release: When your body is properly aligned, you can access deeper stretches and release tension more effectively in targeted areas. By aligning your joints, lengthening your muscles, and engaging in mindful stretching, you unlock tightness, increase flexibility, and experience a greater sense of freedom and ease in your body.

Supports Spinal Health: Maintaining proper posture and alignment is crucial for spinal health and longevity. By aligning your spine in neutral alignment and avoiding excessive rounding or arching, you protect the integrity of your vertebrae, discs, and surrounding structures, reducing the risk of back pain or injury.

Boosts Confidence and Presence: When you embody proper posture and alignment, you exude confidence, poise, and presence—both on and off the mat. By standing tall, lifting your heart, and grounding through your feet, you project an air of strength, vitality, and self-assurance that radiates from within.

Accelerates Weight Loss Results: Last but certainly not least, mastering proper posture and technique accelerates your weight loss results and amplifies the effectiveness of your chair yoga practice. By ensuring that you engage the right muscles, optimize your breath, and move with precision and intention, you maximize calorie burn, build lean muscle mass, and sculpt your body more efficiently.

Remember: in the realm of chair yoga for weight loss, every detail matters, and every adjustment counts. So as you embark on this transformative journey, commit to embracing proper posture and technique with diligence, dedication, and unwavering attention. Your body will thank you, your practice will flourish, and your weight loss goals will become a reality—step by step, pose by pose, breath by breath.

- **Offer suggestions for creating a comfortable and safe practice environment**

Welcome to the sanctuary of your chair yoga practice—a sacred space where safety, comfort, and mindfulness converge to support your journey towards weight loss and well-being. In this chapter, we'll explore essential tips and suggestions for creating a practice environment that nurtures your body, mind, and spirit, ensuring that every moment on the mat is one of joy, empowerment, and safety.

1. **Choose the Right Chair**: Begin by selecting a sturdy, stable chair that provides ample support and allows for proper alignment. Opt for a chair with a flat seat, firm backrest, and no wheels to minimize the risk of tipping or sliding during your practice.

2. **Clear Your Space**: Create a dedicated practice area free from clutter or obstacles that could interfere with your movements. Clear a space around your

chair to ensure that you have room to move safely and comfortably in all directions.

3. **Use Props for Support**: Consider incorporating props such as yoga blocks, blankets, or cushions to enhance your comfort and support during your practice. Use blocks to modify poses or provide additional height and stability, blankets for extra padding and warmth, and cushions for added support and relaxation.

4. **Adjust Your Seating Position**: Position your chair on a non-slip surface to prevent it from sliding during your practice. Situate yourself in the center of the chair with your feet flat on the ground and your knees aligned with your hips for optimal stability and alignment.

5. **Mind Your Posture**: Pay attention to your posture throughout your practice, maintaining a tall, elongated spine and relaxed shoulders. Avoid slouching or leaning too far forward or backward, as this can strain your back and neck muscles.

6. **Listen to Your Body**: Tune into your body's signals and honor your limits during your practice. If you experience any discomfort or pain, gently modify or release the pose, and seek guidance from a qualified instructor if needed.

7. **Stay Hydrated**: Keep a water bottle nearby and hydrate regularly during your practice to support your body's natural detoxification process and maintain optimal energy levels.

8. **Warm Up Properly**: Begin your practice with a gentle warm-up to prepare your body for movement and reduce the risk of injury. Incorporate dynamic stretches, gentle twists, and mindful breathing exercises to awaken your muscles and joints.

9. **Cool Down and Stretch**: Conclude your practice with a soothing cool-down and stretching sequence to promote relaxation, flexibility, and recovery. Focus on gentle stretches that target key muscle groups and promote circulation, such as forward folds, side stretches, and gentle twists.

10. **Practice Mindfulness**: Cultivate a mindset of mindfulness and presence throughout your practice, tuning into the sensations of your body, breath, and thoughts with curiosity and compassion. Allow yourself to fully immerse in the present moment, letting go of distractions and expectations as you move with grace and intention.

By implementing these suggestions and creating a safe, supportive practice environment, you can enjoy the benefits of chair yoga for weight loss with confidence, ease, and peace of mind.

WARM UP EXERCISES

1. Seated Cat-Cow Stretch:

- Sit tall on the edge of your chair with your feet flat on the ground.
- Place your hands on your knees or thighs.
- Inhale as you arch your back, lifting your chest and tilting your pelvis forward (Cow Pose).
- Exhale as you round your spine, tucking your chin to your chest and tilting your pelvis backward (Cat Pose).
- Repeat this fluid movement, synchronizing your breath with each motion, for 8-10 rounds.

Variations:

- For a deeper stretch, extend your arms forward on the inhale and draw them back toward your hips on the exhale.
- If you have wrist or shoulder discomfort, keep your hands resting on your thighs throughout the movement.

Benefits:

- Warms up the spine and stretches the back muscles.
- Improves spinal flexibility and mobility.
- Stimulates digestion and enhances circulation.

2. Chair Forward Fold:

- Sit tall on your chair with your feet hip-width apart.
- Inhale as you lengthen your spine and lift your arms overhead.
- Exhale as you hinge forward from your hips, folding your torso over your thighs and reaching your hands toward the floor (or as far as comfortable).
- Allow your head to relax, releasing any tension in your neck.
- Hold the forward fold for 3-5 deep breaths, focusing on relaxing into the stretch with each exhale.

Variations:

- If reaching the floor is challenging, place your hands on your shins or thighs for support.

- Keep a slight bend in your knees if you feel any discomfort in your lower back or hamstrings.

Benefits:

- Stretches the entire back body, including the spine, hamstrings, and calves.
- Relieves tension in the back and neck.
- Calms the mind and reduces stress.

3. Seated Spinal Twist:

- Sit tall on your chair with your feet flat on the ground.
- Inhale to lengthen your spine, then exhale as you twist your torso to the right, placing your left hand on the outside of your right thigh and your right hand on the back of the chair.
- Keep your gaze over your right shoulder, taking care not to strain your neck.
- Hold the twist for 3-5 breaths, feeling the gentle rotation of your spine with each exhale.

- Inhale to return to center, then repeat on the opposite side.

Variations:

- If reaching the back of the chair is challenging, place your right hand on your left knee and your left hand on the armrest of the chair for support.

Benefits:

- Increases spinal mobility and flexibility.
- Stimulates digestion and detoxification.
- Relieves tension in the spine and shoulders.

4. Seated Knee to Chest Stretch:

- Sit tall on your chair with your feet flat on the ground.
- Inhale to lengthen your spine, then exhale as you lift your right knee toward your chest, wrapping your arms around your shin.
- Hold the stretch for 3-5 breaths, gently drawing your knee closer to your chest with each exhale.

- Release and switch sides, bringing your left knee toward your chest.

Variations:

- If hugging your knee is challenging, place your hands behind your thigh or use a yoga strap looped around your foot for assistance.

Benefits:

- Stretches the hips, thighs, and lower back.
- Improves hip mobility and flexibility.
- Stimulates circulation and releases tension in the lower body.

5. Seated Side Bend:

- Sit tall on your chair with your feet flat on the ground and your hands resting on your thighs.
- Inhale to lengthen your spine, then exhale as you side bend to the right, sliding your right hand down your leg and reaching your left arm overhead.

- Keep both sit bones grounded on the chair and avoid collapsing into the side bend.
- Hold the stretch for 3-5 breaths, feeling a gentle opening along the left side of your body.
- Inhale to return to center, then repeat on the left side.

Variations:

- If reaching the ground is challenging, place your right hand on the armrest of the chair for support as you side bend to the right.

Benefits:

- Stretches the side body, including the intercostal muscles and obliques.
- Improves lateral mobility and flexibility.
- Opens the chest and lungs, enhancing breath capacity.

These warm-up chair yoga exercises will help you prepare your body for your weight loss practice by increasing circulation, improving mobility, and enhancing body awareness. Remember to move mindfully, breathe deeply, and listen to your body's needs as you explore each pose.

EXERCISES

1. Seated Mountain Pose:

- Sit tall on the edge of your chair with your feet flat on the ground and your knees aligned with your hips.

- Place your hands on your thighs with palms facing down.

- Inhale deeply as you lengthen your spine, lifting the crown of your head towards the ceiling.

- Engage your abdominal muscles and press your feet firmly into the ground.

- Hold the pose for 5-10 breaths, focusing on creating length and stability in the spine.

Variations:

- For a deeper stretch, you can reach your arms overhead and interlace your fingers, stretching upwards.

- If you have shoulder issues, you can keep your hands on your thighs or bring them into prayer position at your heart center.

Benefits:

- Improves posture by strengthening the muscles of the back and core.
- Promotes a sense of grounding and stability.
- Increases awareness of breath and body alignment.

2. Seated Chair Twist with Eagle Arms:

- Sit tall on your chair with your feet flat on the ground.
- Cross your right arm under your left arm, wrapping your forearms together and bringing your palms to touch (or as close as possible).
- Inhale to lengthen your spine, then exhale as you twist your torso to the left, hooking your right elbow outside your left thigh.
- Press your palms together to deepen the twist, keeping your spine tall and your shoulders relaxed.
- Hold the twist for 3-5 breaths, feeling the gentle rotation of your spine.

- Inhale to release and switch sides, crossing your left arm under your right arm and twisting to the right.

Variations:

- If you have shoulder issues, you can simply cross your arms in front of your chest without wrapping them together.
- For a deeper stretch, you can lift your elbows slightly and draw your hands away from your face.

Benefits:

- Increases spinal mobility and flexibility, aiding in digestion and detoxification.
- Stretches the muscles of the shoulders, upper back, and chest.
- Engages the core muscles, promoting stability and balance.

3. Seated Warrior III Pose:

- Sit tall on the edge of your chair with your feet hip-width apart and flat on the ground.

- Extend your right leg straight back behind you, flexing your foot and engaging your quadriceps.

- Keep your spine long and your torso parallel to the ground, reaching your arms forward in line with your ears.

- Engage your core muscles to maintain balance, and focus on a point in front of you for stability.

- Hold the pose for 3-5 breaths, feeling the strength and stability in your standing leg.

- Inhale to release and switch sides, extending your left leg straight back behind you.

Variations:

- If balancing on one leg is challenging, you can place your hands on the back of the chair for support.

- For an added challenge, you can lift your extended leg higher, bringing it closer to parallel with the ground.

Benefits:

- Strengthens the muscles of the legs, core, and back.

- Improves balance, coordination, and proprioception.

- Energizes the body and promotes a sense of focus and concentration.

4. Seated Boat Pose:

- Sit tall on your chair with your knees bent and your feet flat on the ground.

- Place your hands on the sides of the chair for support.

- Engage your core muscles and lean back slightly, lifting your feet off the ground and straightening your legs in front of you.

- Keep your spine long and your chest lifted, balancing on your sitting bones.

- Hold the pose for 3-5 breaths, feeling the strength and activation in your abdominal muscles.

- Exhale to release and lower your feet back to the ground.

Variations:

- If lifting both feet off the ground is challenging, you can alternate lifting one foot at a time or keep one foot grounded for stability.
- For an added challenge, you can extend your arms forward in line with your shoulders, palms facing each other.

Benefits:

- Strengthens the muscles of the core, including the abdominals, obliques, and hip flexors.
- Improves posture and spinal alignment.
- Stimulates digestion and metabolism, aiding in weight loss efforts.

5. Seated Leg Extension with Arm Reach:

- Sit tall on your chair with your feet flat on the ground and your hands resting on your thighs.
- Inhale to lengthen your spine, then exhale as you extend your right leg straight out in front of you, engaging your quadriceps.
- At the same time, reach your left arm up and over your head, lengthening through the side body.
- Hold the extended position for a few breaths, feeling the stretch in your hamstring and side body.
- Inhale to release and switch sides, extending your left leg and reaching your right arm up and over.

Variations:

- If reaching overhead is challenging, you can simply reach your arm out to the side or place your hand on your hip.
- For an added challenge, you can pulse your leg up and down or hold the extended position for a longer duration.

Benefits:

- Stretches the hamstrings, calves, and side body, improving flexibility and mobility.
- Strengthens the muscles of the core, shoulders, and arms.
- Promotes balance and coordination, enhancing overall stability and body awareness.

6. Seated Chair Pose (Utkatasana):

- Sit tall on the edge of your chair with your feet hip-width apart and flat on the ground.
- Inhale as you raise your arms overhead, palms facing each other.
- Exhale as you bend your knees and lower your hips toward the chair, as if you're sitting back into an imaginary chair.
- Keep your chest lifted and your spine long, engaging your core muscles to support your lower back.

- Hold the pose for 3-5 breaths, feeling the strength and activation in your legs.

Variations:

- If you have knee issues, you can perform a gentler variation by only bending your knees slightly instead of coming into a full squat position.
- For an added challenge, you can hold small weights in each hand or lift your heels off the ground as you lower into the pose.

Benefits:

- Strengthens the muscles of the legs, glutes, and core.
- Improves lower body endurance and stamina.
- Increases calorie burn and metabolic rate.

7. Seated Side Leg Lifts:

- Sit tall on your chair with your feet flat on the ground and your hands resting on your thighs.

- Inhale to lengthen your spine, then exhale as you lift your right leg out to the side, keeping it straight and engaging your outer thigh.

- Hold the lifted position for a few breaths, then lower your right leg back to the ground.

- Repeat on the left side, lifting and lowering your left leg with control.

- Continue alternating legs for 8-10 repetitions on each side.

Variations:

- If lifting your leg is challenging, you can perform a smaller range of motion or use your hands for support by holding onto the sides of the chair.

- For an added challenge, you can perform the leg lifts with ankle weights or a resistance band wrapped around your thighs.

Benefits:

- Targets the muscles of the outer thighs and hips, helping to tone and sculpt the legs.

- Improves hip mobility and stability.

- Enhances balance and proprioception.

8. Seated Forward Bend with Twist:

- Sit tall on your chair with your feet flat on the ground and your hands resting on your thighs.

- Inhale to lengthen your spine, then exhale as you hinge forward from your hips, folding your torso over your thighs.

- Hold onto the sides of the chair for support as you twist your torso to the right, reaching your left hand towards the outside of your right foot.

- Hold the twist for a few breaths, feeling the stretch along the left side of your body.

- Inhale to release the twist and return to center, then repeat on the left side.

Variations:

- If reaching the foot is challenging, you can place your hand on your shin or thigh instead.
- For a deeper stretch, you can place your opposite hand on the seat of the chair and twist your torso further, looking over your shoulder.

Benefits:

- Stretches the entire back body, including the spine, hamstrings, and side body.
- Stimulates digestion and detoxification, promoting a healthy metabolism.
- Relieves tension in the back, hips, and shoulders.

9. Seated Warrior I Pose:

- Sit tall on your chair with your feet flat on the ground and your hands resting on your thighs.
- Extend your right leg back behind you, bending your knee and planting the ball of your foot on the ground.
- Square your hips towards the front of the chair and engage your core muscles.
- Inhale as you raise your arms overhead, palms facing each other.
- Hold the pose for 3-5 breaths, feeling the strength and stability in your legs and core.
- Exhale to release and switch sides, extending your left leg back and raising your arms overhead.

Variations:

- If balance is challenging, you can hold onto the sides of the chair for support or perform the pose with your back knee resting on the seat of the chair.
- For an added challenge, you can deepen the lunge by bending your front knee further and sinking your hips lower.

Benefits:

- Strengthens the muscles of the legs, core, and arms.

- Improves balance, stability, and proprioception.

- Energizes the body and promotes a sense of empowerment.

10. Seated Chair Twist with Leg Extension:

- Sit tall on your chair with your feet flat on the ground and your hands resting on your thighs.

- Inhale to lengthen your spine, then exhale as you twist your torso to the right, placing your left hand on the outside of your right thigh.

- Extend your right leg out to the side, keeping it straight and engaging your quadriceps.

- Hold the twist and leg extension for a few breaths, feeling the stretch along the spine and inner thigh.

- Inhale to release and return to center, then repeat on the left side.

Variations:

- If extending your leg is challenging, you can keep both feet grounded on the floor or perform the twist without the leg extension.
- For an added challenge, you can reach your opposite arm towards the foot of the extended leg, deepening the twist.

Benefits:

- Increases spinal mobility and flexibility.
- Stretches the muscles of the inner thigh and groin.
- Engages the core muscles, promoting stability and balance.

11.   Seated Warrior I Pose:

- Sit tall on your chair with your feet flat on the ground and your hands resting on your thighs.

- Extend your right leg back behind you, keeping it straight, and press the ball of your foot into the ground.

- Bend your left knee, bringing it directly over your left ankle, and keep your torso upright.

- Inhale as you reach your arms overhead, bringing your palms together.

- Gaze forward and hold the pose for 3-5 breaths, feeling the strength and stability in your legs and core.

- Exhale to release and switch sides, extending your left leg back and bending your right knee.

Variations:

- If you have limited space or balance, you can perform a seated variation by simply reaching your arms overhead while seated in the chair.

Benefits:

- Strengthens the muscles of the legs, core, and arms.
- Improves balance and stability, promoting better posture and alignment.
- Energizes the body and stimulates circulation.

12. Seated Side Bend with Arm Reach:

- Sit tall on your chair with your feet flat on the ground and your hands resting on your thighs.
- Inhale deeply as you reach your right arm up and over your head, lengthening through the side body.
- Exhale as you lean to the left, stretching through the right side of your torso.
- Hold the stretch for a few breaths, feeling the lengthening sensation along the right side of your body.
- Inhale to return to center, then repeat on the opposite side.

Variations:

- For a deeper stretch, you can hold onto the side of the chair with your left hand and lean further into the side bend.
- If reaching overhead is challenging, you can simply reach your arm out to the side or place your hand on your hip.

Benefits:

- Stretches the muscles of the side body, including the intercostal muscles and obliques.
- Improves spinal mobility and flexibility, reducing tension and stiffness in the back.
- Promotes better posture and alignment, enhancing overall body awareness.

13.   Seated High Knees:

- Sit tall on your chair with your feet flat on the ground and your hands resting on your thighs.

- Engage your core muscles and lift your right knee towards your chest as high as comfortable.

- Hold the lifted position for a few seconds, then lower your right foot back to the ground.

- Repeat on the left side, lifting and lowering your left knee with control.

- Continue alternating legs for 8-10 repetitions on each side.

Variations:

- For an added challenge, you can increase the speed of the movement, performing quick high knee lifts to elevate the heart rate.

- If lifting both knees simultaneously is challenging, you can focus on one leg at a time or perform a marching motion, lifting one knee at a time.

Benefits:

- Strengthens the muscles of the core, including the abdominals and hip flexors.

- Increases heart rate and calorie burn, supporting weight loss efforts.

- Improves coordination and balance, promoting better functional movement patterns.

14. Seated Crescent Moon Stretch:

- Sit tall on your chair with your feet flat on the ground and your hands resting on your thighs.

- Inhale deeply as you reach your arms overhead, clasping your hands together.

- Lean gently to the right, creating a side stretch along the left side of your body.

- Hold the stretch for a few breaths, feeling the lengthening sensation along the left side.

- Inhale to return to center, then exhale as you lean to the left, stretching through the right side of your body.

Variations:

- For a deeper stretch, you can hold onto the side of the chair with one hand while reaching overhead with the other.

- If reaching overhead is challenging, you can simply reach your arms out to the sides or place your hands on your hips.

Benefits:

- Stretches the muscles of the side body, including the obliques and intercostal muscles.

- Increases flexibility and mobility in the spine, reducing tension and stiffness.

- Promotes better posture and alignment, enhancing overall body awareness.

15. Seated Leg Cross with Forward Fold:

- Sit tall on your chair with your feet flat on the ground and your hands resting on your thighs.

- Cross your right ankle over your left knee, flexing your right foot to protect the knee joint.

- Inhale to lengthen your spine, then exhale as you hinge forward from your hips, folding your torso over your crossed leg.

- Hold the forward fold for a few breaths, feeling the stretch in your right outer hip and glute.

- Inhale to return to an upright position, then switch sides, crossing your left ankle over your right knee and folding forward.

Variations:

- For a deeper stretch, you can place your hands on the floor in front of you and walk them forward, lowering your chest towards your shin.

- If folding forward is challenging, you can simply sit upright and gently press down on your crossed knee to deepen the stretch.

Benefits:

- Stretches the muscles of the outer hips and glutes, reducing tension and discomfort.

- Improves flexibility and mobility in the hip joints, promoting better range of motion.

- Relieves sciatic nerve pain and discomfort associated with prolonged sitting.

16.   Seated Twist with Leg Extension:

- Sit tall on your chair with your feet flat on the ground and your hands resting on your thighs.

- Inhale deeply as you lengthen your spine, then exhale as you twist your torso to the right, placing your left hand on your right knee.

- Extend your right leg straight out in front of you, keeping it parallel to the ground.

- Hold the twist for a few breaths, feeling the gentle rotation of your spine.

- Inhale to return to center, then repeat on the opposite side, twisting to the left and extending your left leg.

Variations:

- For a deeper twist, you can hook your elbow over the opposite knee and press your palms together in prayer position.

- If extending your leg is challenging, you can keep both feet flat on the ground and focus on the seated twist.

Benefits:

- Increases spinal mobility and flexibility, reducing stiffness and discomfort in the back.

- Stretches the muscles of the hips, hamstrings, and glutes, improving flexibility and range of motion.

- Stimulates digestion and detoxification, promoting a healthy metabolism.

17. Seated Chair Pigeon Pose:

- Sit tall on your chair with your feet flat on the ground and your hands resting on your thighs.

- Cross your right ankle over your left knee, flexing your right foot to protect the knee joint.

- Keep your spine long and your chest lifted as you gently press down on your right knee, opening up the right hip.

- Hold the stretch for a few breaths, feeling the sensation in your right outer hip and glute.

- Inhale to release and switch sides, crossing your left ankle over your right knee.

Variations:

- For a deeper stretch, you can hinge forward from your hips, folding your torso over your crossed leg.

- If crossing your ankle over your knee is challenging, you can simply place your ankle on top of your thigh and press down gently on your knee.

Benefits:

- Stretches the muscles of the outer hips and glutes, reducing tension and discomfort.

- Opens up the hip joint, improving flexibility and mobility.

- Relieves sciatic nerve pain and discomfort associated with prolonged sitting.

18.   Seated   Wide-Legged Forward Fold:

- Sit tall on your chair with your feet wider than hip-width apart and your toes pointing forward.

- Inhale deeply as you lengthen your spine, then exhale as you hinge forward from your hips, folding your torso forward.

- Keep your spine long and your chest lifted as you reach your hands towards the ground (or as far as comfortable).

- Hold the forward fold for a few breaths, feeling the stretch along the inner thighs and hamstrings.

- Inhale to return to an upright position, then exhale as you gently release the stretch.

Variations:

- For a deeper stretch, you can walk your hands forward between your legs and lower your chest towards the ground.

- If reaching the ground is challenging, you can place your hands on yoga blocks or books for support.

Benefits:

- Stretches the muscles of the inner thighs, hamstrings, and groin, reducing tension and stiffness.

- Improves flexibility and mobility in the hip joints, promoting better range of motion.

- Stimulates digestion and detoxification, supporting a healthy metabolism.

19. Seated Knee-to-Chest Twist:

- Sit tall on your chair with your feet flat on the ground and your hands resting on your thighs.

- Inhale deeply as you lift your right knee towards your chest, hugging it with both hands.

- Exhale as you gently twist your torso to the right, bringing your right knee across your body towards your left shoulder.

- Hold the twist for a few breaths, feeling the stretch in your lower back and outer hip.

- Inhale to release and switch sides, bringing your left knee towards your chest and twisting to the left.

Variations:

- For a deeper stretch, you can hook your elbow over the opposite knee and press your palms together in prayer position.

- If hugging your knee is challenging, you can place your hands behind your thigh for support.

Benefits:

- Increases spinal mobility and flexibility, reducing stiffness and discomfort in the back.

- Stretches the muscles of the lower back, hips, and glutes, relieving tension and discomfort.

- Stimulates digestion and detoxification, promoting a healthy metabolism.

20. Seated Eagle Arms with Forward Fold:

- Sit tall on your chair with your feet flat on the ground and your hands resting on your thighs.

- Inhale deeply as you reach your arms out to the sides, parallel to the ground.

- Exhale as you cross your right arm under your left arm, wrapping your forearms together and bringing your palms to touch.

- Lift your elbows slightly and press your palms together, feeling the stretch in your shoulders and upper back.

- Inhale to lengthen your spine, then exhale as you hinge forward from your hips, folding your torso over your crossed arms.

- Hold the forward fold for a few breaths, feeling the stretch in your upper back and shoulders.

Variations:

- If crossing your arms is challenging, you can simply reach your arms out to the sides or place your hands on your shoulders.

- For a deeper stretch, you can lift your elbows higher and press your palms together more firmly.

Benefits:

- Stretches the muscles of the shoulders, upper back, and chest, reducing tension and stiffness.

- Improves posture and spinal alignment, promoting better body awareness and alignment.

- Relieves stress and tension in the upper body, promoting relaxation and calm.

21.   Seated Chair Twist with Leg Cross:

- Sit tall on your chair with your feet flat on the ground and your hands resting on your thighs.

- Inhale deeply as you lengthen your spine, then exhale as you twist your torso to the right, placing your left hand on the outside of your right thigh.

- Cross your right ankle over your left knee, flexing your right foot to protect the knee joint.

- Hold the twist for a few breaths, feeling the gentle rotation of your spine and the stretch in your outer hip.

- Inhale to return to center, then exhale as you twist to the left and cross your left ankle over your right knee.

Variations:

- For a deeper twist, you can hook your elbow over the opposite knee and press your palms together in prayer position.

- If crossing your ankle over your knee is challenging, you can simply place your ankle on top of your thigh and press down gently on your knee.

Benefits:

- Increases spinal mobility and flexibility, reducing stiffness and discomfort in the back.

- Stretches the muscles of the outer hips and glutes, relieving tension and discomfort.

- Promotes better posture and alignment, enhancing overall body awareness.

22. Seated Warrior III with Leg Lift:

- Sit tall on your chair with your feet flat on the ground and your hands resting on your thighs.

- Inhale deeply as you lengthen your spine, then exhale as you hinge forward from your hips, bringing your torso parallel to the ground.

- Extend your right leg straight back behind you, keeping it parallel to the ground and your foot flexed.

- Engage your core muscles and lift your right leg a few inches higher, feeling the activation in your glutes and hamstrings.

- Hold the lifted position for a few breaths, then lower your right leg back to the ground.

- Repeat on the left side, extending your left leg straight back and lifting it a few inches off the ground.

Variations:

- If lifting your leg is challenging, you can keep both feet on the ground and focus on maintaining a flat back in the seated forward fold.

- For an added challenge, you can extend your arms forward in line with your ears, creating a straight line from your fingertips to your extended heel.

Benefits:

- Strengthens the muscles of the core, glutes, and hamstrings, promoting better posture and stability.

- Improves balance and proprioception, enhancing overall body awareness and coordination.

- Increases calorie burn and metabolic rate, supporting weight loss efforts.

23. Seated Side Plank:

- Sit tall on your chair with your feet flat on the ground and your hands resting on your thighs.

- Place your right hand on the seat of the chair, directly underneath your shoulder.

- Inhale deeply as you engage your core muscles, then exhale as you lift your hips off the chair, coming into a side plank position.

- Extend your left arm overhead, reaching towards the ceiling, and stack your feet or stagger them for stability.

- Hold the side plank for a few breaths, feeling the activation in your obliques and outer hip.

- Inhale to lower your hips back to the chair, then repeat on the opposite side.

Variations:

- If lifting your hips off the chair is challenging, you can simply hold a static side plank with your hips resting on the chair.

- For an added challenge, you can lift your top leg towards the ceiling or perform hip dips, lowering and lifting your hips in a controlled motion.

Benefits:

- Strengthens the muscles of the core, shoulders, and arms, promoting better posture and stability.

- Improves balance and proprioception, enhancing overall body awareness and coordination.

- Increases calorie burn and metabolic rate, supporting weight loss efforts.

24. Seated Boat Pose:

- Sit tall on your chair with your feet flat on the ground and your hands resting on your thighs.

- Engage your core muscles and lean back slightly, lifting your feet off the ground.

- Extend your legs straight out in front of you, keeping them parallel to the ground.

- Hold the pose for 5-10 breaths, maintaining a straight spine and lifted chest.

- To release, gently lower your feet back to the ground.

Variations:

- For an added challenge, you can extend your arms forward alongside your legs or reach them overhead.

- If lifting both feet simultaneously is challenging, you can alternate lifting one foot at a time.

Benefits:

- Strengthens the core muscles, including the abdominals and lower back.

- Improves balance and stability, promoting better posture and body awareness.

- Increases calorie burn and supports weight loss efforts.

25. Seated Leg Extension with Twist:

- Sit tall on your chair with your feet flat on the ground and your hands resting on your thighs.

- Inhale deeply as you extend your right leg straight out in front of you.

- Exhale as you twist your torso to the right, bringing your left hand to the outside of your right knee.

- Hold the twist for a few breaths, feeling the stretch in your spine and outer hip.

- Inhale to return to center, then switch sides, extending your left leg and twisting to the left.

Variations:

- For a deeper stretch, you can hook your elbow over the opposite knee and press your palms together in prayer position.

- If extending your leg is challenging, you can simply focus on the seated twist without the leg extension.

Benefits:

- Increases spinal mobility and flexibility, reducing stiffness and discomfort.

- Stretches the muscles of the hips, hamstrings, and lower back, promoting better range of motion.

- Improves digestion and detoxification, supporting weight loss efforts.

26. Seated Mountain Pose with Arm Circles:

- Sit tall on your chair with your feet flat on the ground and your hands resting on your thighs.

- Inhale deeply as you reach your arms out to the sides, parallel to the ground.

- Exhale as you circle your arms forward in small circles, moving from the shoulders.

- Continue circling your arms for 10-15 repetitions, then reverse the direction and circle them backward.

- Focus on keeping your spine tall and your breath steady throughout the movement.

Variations:

- You can perform larger circles with your arms for a deeper shoulder stretch and more dynamic movement.

- If sitting upright is challenging, you can lean back slightly in the chair for added support.

Benefits:

- Improves shoulder mobility and flexibility, reducing tension and stiffness in the upper body.

- Increases circulation and blood flow to the arms and shoulders, promoting a sense of energy and vitality.

- Enhances body awareness and mindfulness, supporting overall well-being and weight loss efforts.

27. Seated Figure Four Stretch:

- Sit tall on your chair with your feet flat on the ground and your hands resting on your thighs.

- Lift your right foot off the ground and cross your right ankle over your left knee, flexing your right foot to protect the knee joint.

- Inhale deeply as you lengthen your spine, then exhale as you hinge forward from your hips, bringing your chest towards your crossed leg.

- Hold the stretch for 5-10 breaths, feeling the sensation in your right outer hip and glute.

- Inhale to release and switch sides, crossing your left ankle over your right knee and folding forward.

Variations:

- For a deeper stretch, you can press gently down on your crossed knee with your hand to increase the stretch in your hip.

- If folding forward is challenging, you can simply sit upright and focus on pressing your knee gently towards the ground.

Benefits:

- Stretches the muscles of the outer hips and glutes, reducing tension and discomfort.

- Improves hip mobility and flexibility, promoting better range of motion and ease of movement.

- Relieves sciatic nerve pain and discomfort associated with prolonged sitting, supporting overall comfort and well-being.

28. Seated Spinal Twist with Leg Extension:

- Sit tall on your chair with your feet flat on the ground and your hands resting on your thighs.

- Inhale deeply as you lengthen your spine, then exhale as you twist your torso to the right, bringing your left hand to the outside of your right knee.

- Extend your right leg straight out in front of you, keeping it parallel to the ground.

- Hold the twist for 5-10 breaths, feeling the stretch in your spine and outer hip.

- Inhale to release and switch sides, twisting to the left and extending your left leg.

Variations:

- For a deeper twist, you can hook your elbow over the opposite knee and press your palms together in prayer position.

- If extending your leg is challenging, you can simply focus on the seated twist without the leg extension.

Benefits:

- Increases spinal mobility and flexibility, reducing stiffness and discomfort in the back.

- Stretches the muscles of the hips, hamstrings, and lower back, promoting better range of motion.

- Stimulates digestion and detoxification, supporting weight loss efforts.

29. Seated Forward Bend with Twist:

- Sit tall on your chair with your feet flat on the ground and your hands resting on your thighs.

- Inhale deeply as you lengthen your spine, then exhale as you hinge forward from your hips, folding your torso over your thighs.

- Once folded forward, place your right hand on the outside of your left knee.

- Inhale to lengthen your spine, and as you exhale, twist your torso to the left, looking over your left shoulder.

- Hold the twist for a few breaths, feeling the stretch along your spine and the outer hip.

- Inhale to release the twist, then repeat on the opposite side, placing your left hand on the outside of your right knee and twisting to the right.

Benefits:

- Stretches the spine, shoulders, and hips.

- Stimulates digestion and detoxification.

- Releases tension in the back and neck.

30.   Seated Leg Raises:

- Sit tall on your chair with your feet flat on the ground and your hands resting on your thighs.

- Engage your core muscles and extend your right leg out in front of you, keeping it straight.

- Inhale as you lift your right leg as high as comfortable, keeping your foot flexed.

- Exhale as you lower your right leg back down to the ground.

- Repeat the leg raises with your right leg for several repetitions, then switch to your left leg.

Benefits:

- Strengthens the muscles of the core, quadriceps, and hip flexors.

- Increases circulation and blood flow to the lower body.

- Improves balance and stability.

31.   Seated Side Stretch:

- Sit tall on your chair with your feet flat on the ground and your hands resting on your thighs.

- Inhale deeply as you lengthen your spine, then exhale as you reach your right arm overhead, leaning to the left.

- Keep your left hand on your left thigh for support and avoid collapsing into the stretch.

- Hold the stretch for a few breaths, feeling the lengthening sensation along the right side of your body.

- Inhale to return to center, then repeat on the opposite side.

Benefits:

- Stretches the muscles of the side body, including the obliques and intercostal muscles.

- Improves spinal mobility and flexibility.

- Promotes better posture and alignment.

32.   Seated Chair Twist with Arm Reach:

- Sit tall on your chair with your feet flat on the ground and your hands resting on your thighs.

- Inhale deeply as you lengthen your spine, then exhale as you twist your torso to the right, placing your left hand on your right knee.

- Reach your right arm behind you, placing your hand on the back of the chair for support.

- Inhale to lengthen your spine, then exhale as you twist further, reaching your right arm up towards the ceiling.

- Hold the twist for a few breaths, feeling the rotation in your spine and the stretch in your chest and shoulders.

- Inhale to release and return to center, then repeat on the opposite side.

Benefits:

- Increases spinal mobility and flexibility.

- Stretches the muscles of the chest, shoulders, and upper back.

- Improves circulation and blood flow.

33. Seated Chair Mountain Pose (Tadasana):

- Sit tall on your chair with your feet flat on the ground and your hands resting on your thighs.

- Inhale deeply as you lengthen your spine, lifting your arms overhead with your palms facing each other.

- Engage your core muscles and press firmly into your feet, feeling the connection to the ground.

- Hold the pose for a few breaths, lengthening through your spine and reaching towards the ceiling.

- Keep your shoulders relaxed and your gaze forward, maintaining steady breathing throughout the pose.

Benefits:

- Improves posture and alignment.

- Increases energy and vitality.

- Promotes a sense of grounding and stability.

These chair yoga exercises offer a variety of movements to target different muscle groups, improve flexibility, and promote circulation, all of which contribute to weight loss and overall well-being.

28-DAYS CHAIR YOGA FOR WEIGHT LOSS CHALLENGE

Day 1: Introduction to Chair Yoga

- Morning: Begin with 5 minutes of deep breathing exercises while seated in your chair.

- Afternoon: Practice Seated Mountain Pose (Tadasana) for 5 minutes, focusing on grounding and elongating the spine.

- Evening: End the day with a 5-minute seated meditation, focusing on relaxation and releasing tension.

Day 2: Core Activation

- Morning: Perform Seated Knee-to-Chest Crunches for 5 minutes to engage the core muscles.

- Afternoon: Practice Seated Side Bend with Arm Reach for 5 minutes on each side to stretch the side body.

- Evening: End with 5 minutes of Seated Boat Pose (Navasana) to further strengthen the core muscles.

Day 3: Lower Body Stretch

- Morning: Perform Seated Forward Fold for 5 minutes to stretch the hamstrings and lower back.

- Afternoon: Practice Seated Pigeon Pose for 5 minutes on each side to open up the hips and release tension.

- Evening: End with 5 minutes of Seated Wide-Legged Forward Fold to stretch the inner thighs and groins.

Day 4: Upper Body Strength

- Morning: Perform Seated Eagle Arms with Forward Fold for 5 minutes to strengthen the arms and shoulders.

- Afternoon: Practice Seated Cat-Cow Stretch for 5 minutes to mobilize the spine and strengthen the core.

- Evening: End with 5 minutes of Seated Shoulder Opener to release tension in the shoulders and upper back.

Day 5: Balance and Stability

- Morning: Perform Seated Warrior III for 5 minutes on each leg to improve balance and stability.

- Afternoon: Practice Seated Tree Pose for 5 minutes on each leg to further enhance balance and focus.

- Evening: End with 5 minutes of Seated Half Moon Pose to stretch the sides of the body and improve overall stability.

Day 6: Flexibility Focus

- Morning: Start with 5 minutes of Seated Forward Bend with Twist to stretch the hamstrings and spine.

- Afternoon: Practice Seated Butterfly Stretch for 5 minutes to open up the hips and inner thighs.

- Evening: End with 5 minutes of Seated Spinal Twist on each side to release tension in the back and improve spinal mobility.

Day 7: Mindful Movement

- Morning: Perform Seated Sun Salutation for 5 minutes, linking breath with movement to energize the body.

- Afternoon: Practice Seated Warrior Flow for 5 minutes, moving fluidly between Warrior I, II, and III poses.

- Evening: End with 5 minutes of Seated Meditation, focusing on mindfulness and cultivating inner peace.

Day 8: Strength and Stability

- Morning: Perform Seated Chair Pose (Utkatasana) for 5 minutes to strengthen the legs and core.

- Afternoon: Practice Seated Plank Pose for 5 minutes to engage the core muscles and improve stability.

- Evening: End with 5 minutes of Seated Side Plank on each side to further enhance core strength and stability.

Day 9: Energizing Flow

- Morning: Start with 5 minutes of Seated Mountain Pose with Arm Variation to energize the body and focus the mind.

- Afternoon: Practice Seated Warrior Flow with Chair for 5 minutes, flowing between Warrior I, II, and III poses.

- Evening: End with 5 minutes of Seated Backbend to open up the chest and improve posture.

Day 10: Stress Relief

- Morning: Perform Seated Forward Fold with Relaxation for 5 minutes to release tension in the back and shoulders.

- Afternoon: Practice Seated Heart Opener for 5 minutes to open up the chest and cultivate a sense of openness.

- Evening: End with 5 minutes of Seated Relaxation Pose to promote deep relaxation and stress relief.

Day 11: Core Strength

- Morning: Start with 5 minutes of Seated Boat Pose (Navasana) to strengthen the core muscles.

- Afternoon: Practice Seated Leg Raises for 5 minutes, lifting and lowering the legs to engage the abdominal muscles.

- Evening: End with 5 minutes of Seated Side Crunches on each side to further target the obliques.

Day 12: Balance Challenge

- Morning: Perform Seated Half Moon Pose for 5 minutes on each side to challenge balance and focus.

- Afternoon: Practice Seated Tree Pose with Arm Variation for 5 minutes on each leg to further enhance balance and stability.

- Evening: End with 5 minutes of Seated Warrior III
  with Leg Lift on each leg to improve balance and
  core strength.

Day 13: Flexibility Flow

- Morning: Start with 5 minutes of Seated Forward
  Bend with Twist to stretch the hamstrings and
  spine.

- Afternoon: Practice Seated Wide-Legged Forward
  Fold for 5 minutes to open up the hips and inner
  thighs.

- Evening: End with 5 minutes of Seated Butterfly
  Stretch to release tension in the hips and lower
  back.

Day 14: Rest and Restore

- Morning: Perform 5 minutes of gentle Seated Cat-
  Cow Stretch to warm up the spine and release
  tension.

- Afternoon: Practice 5 minutes of Seated Neck and
  Shoulder Release to relax and unwind tight muscles.

- Evening: End with 5 minutes of Seated Breathing Meditation to promote deep relaxation and inner peace.

Day 15: Strength and Flexibility

- Morning: Perform Seated Warrior II Pose for 5 minutes on each side to strengthen the legs and open up the hips.

- Afternoon: Practice Seated Extended Side Angle Pose for 5 minutes on each side to stretch the side body and improve flexibility.

- Evening: End with 5 minutes of Seated Revolved Head-to-Knee Pose on each side to stretch the spine and hamstrings.

Day 16: Core Stability

- Morning: Start with 5 minutes of Seated Boat Pose (Navasana) to engage the core muscles and improve balance.

- Afternoon: Practice Seated Side Plank with Leg Lift for 5 minutes on each side to further challenge core stability and strength.

- Evening: End with 5 minutes of Seated Russian Twists to target the obliques and improve rotational strength.

Day 17: Hip Opening

- Morning: Perform Seated Pigeon Pose for 5 minutes on each side to open up the hips and release tension.

- Afternoon: Practice Seated Hip Opener for 5 minutes on each side to further stretch the hips and inner thighs.

- Evening: End with 5 minutes of Seated Butterfly Stretch to relax and release tension in the hips and groin.

Day 18: Balance and Focus

- Morning: Start with 5 minutes of Seated Tree Pose on each leg to improve balance and focus.

- Afternoon: Practice Seated Warrior III Pose for 5 minutes on each leg to challenge balance and strengthen the core.

- Evening: End with 5 minutes of Seated Eagle Pose on each side to further enhance balance and focus.

Day 19: Back Strength

- Morning: Perform Seated Cat-Cow Stretch for 5 minutes to warm up the spine and improve flexibility.

- Afternoon: Practice Seated Cobra Pose for 5 minutes to strengthen the back muscles and improve posture.

- Evening: End with 5 minutes of Seated Locust Pose to further strengthen the back muscles and improve spinal alignment.

Day 20: Full Body Flow

- Morning: Start with 5 minutes of Seated Sun Salutation to warm up the body and energize the mind.

- Afternoon: Practice Seated Warrior Flow for 5 minutes, flowing between Warrior I, II, and III poses to build strength and flexibility.

- Evening: End with 5 minutes of Seated Moon Salutation to calm the mind and relax the body.

Day 21: Core Challenge

- Morning: Perform Seated Knee-to-Chest Crunches for 5 minutes to engage the core muscles and improve abdominal strength.

- Afternoon: Practice Seated Boat Pose (Navasana) for 5 minutes to further challenge core stability and balance.

- Evening: End with 5 minutes of Seated Plank Pose to strengthen the core muscles and improve overall stability.

Day 22: Hip Flexibility

- Morning: Start with 5 minutes of Seated Forward Fold to stretch the hamstrings and lower back.

- Afternoon: Practice Seated Garland Pose for 5 minutes to open up the hips and improve hip flexibility.

- Evening: End with 5 minutes of Seated Wide-Legged Forward Fold to further stretch the inner thighs and groins.

Day 23: Balance Challenge

- Morning: Perform Seated Warrior III Pose for 5 minutes on each leg to challenge balance and strengthen the core.

- Afternoon: Practice Seated Tree Pose with Arm Variation for 5 minutes on each leg to further enhance balance and focus.

- Evening: End with 5 minutes of Seated Half Moon Pose to improve balance and stability while stretching the side body.

Day 24: Strength and Stability

- Morning: Start with 5 minutes of Seated Chair Pose (Utkatasana) to strengthen the legs and core.

- Afternoon: Practice Seated Side Plank for 5 minutes on each side to further challenge core stability and strength.

- Evening: End with 5 minutes of Seated Warrior II Pose to strengthen the legs and improve hip mobility.

Day 25: Flexibility Flow

- Morning: Perform Seated Forward Bend with Twist for 5 minutes to stretch the hamstrings and spine.

- Afternoon: Practice Seated Wide-Legged Forward Fold for 5 minutes to open up the hips and inner thighs.

- Evening: End with 5 minutes of Seated Butterfly Stretch to release tension in the hips and lower back.

Day 26: Mindful Movement

- Morning: Start with 5 minutes of Seated Sun Salutation to energize the body and focus the mind.

- Afternoon: Practice Seated Warrior Flow for 5 minutes, flowing between Warrior I, II, and III poses to build strength and flexibility.

- Evening: End with 5 minutes of Seated Meditation to cultivate mindfulness and inner peace.

Day 27: Strength and Flexibility

- Morning: Perform Seated Warrior II Pose for 5 minutes on each side to strengthen the legs and open up the hips.

- Afternoon: Practice Seated Extended Side Angle Pose for 5 minutes on each side to stretch the side body and improve flexibility.

- Evening: End with 5 minutes of Seated Revolved Head-to-Knee Pose on each side to stretch the spine and hamstrings.

Day 28: Celebration and Reflection

- Morning: Start with 5 minutes of gentle stretching to wake up the body and prepare for the day ahead.

- Afternoon: Reflect on your chair yoga journey and celebrate your achievements over the past 28 days.

- Evening: End with 5 minutes of relaxation and gratitude, expressing appreciation for yourself and your commitment to health and well-being.

Congratulations on completing the 28-day chair yoga challenge!

CONCLUSION

Congratulations, dear reader, on embarking on this transformative journey towards wellness through chair yoga. As we conclude this book, I want to take a moment to express my deepest gratitude for joining me on this path of self-discovery and empowerment.

Throughout these pages, we've explored the incredible benefits of chair yoga for weight loss and overall well-being. From gentle stretches to dynamic flows, each pose and exercise was carefully curated to support you on your quest for a healthier, happier life. But beyond the physical practice lies a profound opportunity for growth, resilience, and self-love.

I want you to know that this journey hasn't been easy for me either. I've faced my own challenges, encountered moments of doubt, and stumbled along the way. But through perseverance, dedication, and a steadfast belief in the power of chair yoga, I've discovered a strength within myself that I never knew existed.

And so, I encourage you to face your journey head-on, with courage, determination, and an unwavering commitment to your well-being. Embrace the ups and downs, celebrate your successes, and learn from your setbacks. Remember that every step you take, no matter how small, brings you closer to your goals.

As you continue your practice beyond these pages, I urge you to cultivate self-compassion and kindness towards yourself. Listen to your body, honor your limitations, and celebrate your progress, no matter how incremental it may seem. Trust in the wisdom of your own inner guidance, and know that you are capable of achieving greatness.

But above all, never forget that you are not alone on this journey. Draw strength from the support of loved ones, seek guidance from experienced practitioners, and find solace in the collective energy of our global community. Together, we can inspire, uplift, and empower one another to reach new heights of health and vitality.

So, as you close this book and step into the world, may you carry with you the wisdom, strength, and courage you've cultivated on the mat. May you embrace each day as an opportunity for growth, and may you continue to shine brightly as the radiant being of light that you are.